Hatha Yoga

*The Ultimate Guide to Mastering Hatha Yoga for Life in 30
Minutes or Less!*

Table of Contents

Introduction

I want to thank you for downloading the book, *"Hatha Yoga: The Ultimate Guide to Mastering Hatha Yoga for Life"*.

In this book you can expect to learn the proven steps and strategies for mastering Hatha Yoga. You may have heard about hatha yoga from your neighbors advocating for and persuading you about it. Whether you are someone who doesn't know anything about it or someone who are already knowledgeable about hatha yoga, this book is for you as it will teach you to become intimately familiar with what hatha yoga truly is including its benefits and how you can reap them. This is the ultimate guide towards doing the yoga poses that you never think you are capable of executing.

If you take the time to read this book fully and apply the information held within this book, it will help you to start a hatha yoga session on your own and in your very own home. You wouldn't even need to pay a yoga instructor a couple of bucks anymore and sign yourself up for weekly sessions because by the end of this book, you will be equipped with the knowledge that you can carry through-out your life.

Thanks again for downloading this book, I hope you enjoy it!

Chapter 1   Hatha Yoga is Not Just Another Indian Fad

Perhaps you're the person who's not so crazy about the mainstream. You observe while people get in line for the next hot thing. For example, you see studios sprouting wherever you go. Across the street, a space is being refurbished to become the new nest for some enthusiasts. And then you find out that yoga is the main event. More and more people that you know have started joining the craze and spending their free times on their heads, doing dog poses and warrior stances you don't have any idea of. You decide to try it for yourself and see what the buzz is all about.

Or perhaps you're the kind of person who has always been up to date. You know what yoga is about and how it can benefit your life. You have always wanted to take a shot of yoga may it be for a change in lifestyle or whatnot.

Either way, this book is for you. It can teach you how to master a type of yoga – hatha yoga – on your own. You see, the problems facing people who want to attempt any form of yoga are various. For one, they don't have sufficient amount of funds to sustain weekly yoga classes. They have enough money to live by and can't afford paying a studio to accommodate them. There's also the issue of time constraints. A busy and hectic study or work schedule doesn't allow for a lot of time for one to sign-up to a studio and do sessions. Because of these reasons, people end up dismissing the idea of doing yoga. But these same reasons shouldn't stop you for you can actually master yoga for life.

There is a lot of yoga styles that you can choose to delve in. And hatha yoga is one of the most popular and prevalent type of yoga being taught across countries. In fact, nearly every type of yoga taught in class in the West is actually hatha yoga. Unlike other forms of yoga, it is a less forceful form of yoga that will gently introduce you to the most basic yoga postures.

Hatha literally means forceful or willful. Hatha yoga is a set of physical exercises and sequences of postures – known as asanas –

that are designed to have your muscles, bones, and skin in alignment. It aims to increase the ability of your body to tolerate stress through making it forcefully undergo different kinds of physical strain. Additionally, it also aims to intensify the endurance of your mind. The asanas or postures are also intended to trigger the opening of the channels in your body, most especially the main channel at your spine, in order for energy to flow freely and uninhibited.

The *ha* from hatha means sun and *tha* means moon. This kind of yoga promotes the balance of both the masculine – personified by the sun which is hot and active – and feminine – represented by the moon which is cool and receptive – aspects that dwell within us. Hatha yoga advocates the union of these opposite aspects, learning how to equalize flexibility and strength.

Hatha yoga is not just another Indian fad as one might immediately think hearing its name but instead, it is a powerful method for self-transformation. After mastering hatha yoga, a better and more disciplined you will emerge.

There are core practices that hatha yoga is composed of. Chanting, for example, is one of them. Saying the word *om* is said to facilitate increase of the yogi's awareness of the present, himself, and the world around him.

Another core practice is *pranayama* or what is known as breath control. Breathing is a vital component of hatha yoga and it is one of the things you must properly do during asanas. Breathing properly will allow energy to flow into the different channels in your body and would provide vitality.

Asanas or postures are the main element of hatha yoga that you must master. Their purpose is to achieve the improvement of physical strength, discipline, balance, and stamina. A sequence of asanas is executed during a hatha yoga session. It must be noted that asanas must be performed in comfort and should never cause pain. In the case of asanas leading to extreme shaking of muscles and unstable breathing, a yogi must stop for he is exerting too much effort and is pushing his body too hard.

Chapter 2   Twist and Turn to See the Benefits

One of the major reasons why people have opted to live a life with yoga in it is the package of benefits that it provides especially health-wise. Hatha yoga, together with other kinds of yoga, provides both therapeutic and preventative health benefits for the mind and body. For people who are opting for a healthier lifestyle, including hatha yoga in their daily menu is a good step to take because of all the mental and physical advantages that it can give.

Some of the physical benefits that hatha yoga can offer include the building of strength. Through the postures or asanas that you will perform, your body will soon get stronger. At the start of your sessions, you may moan about how you can't do any of the asanas but as time goes on and as more yoga sessions that will take place; you will notice that you are already capable of the asanas that you have never executed at the start. Your muscles will then be toned and you will experience an improvement in flexibility and mobility of your muscle joints.

For people who have problems with their postures, hatha yoga is a great way to correct them as it is proven to treat scoliosis, strengthens your spine, and improves tight shoulders and neck, among others.

Hatha yoga will also increase your stamina through the various exercises that will make you exert physical effort. It has also been implicated in the improvement of digestion, blood circulation, and respiration. It can even be an effective method for losing weight.

Moreover, the meditation and breathing exercises involved in hatha yoga will go a long way in reducing accumulated stress. One yoga session could be your time to wind down and dismiss daily dilemmas and annoyances. The mere engagement in the asanas will give you a sense of calm and peace since you are not thinking of anything else that could provide you discomfort.

It teaches you how to sharpen your focus and concentration, how to relax your mind and body from distracting thoughts and unnecessary tension.

Additionally, hatha yoga has been considered by a lot of people as an alternative to exercise. There are even pieces of evidence showing how it can be better compared to strenuous physical exercise.

One of its most distinguishing points of difference from other kinds of exercise is how it's not limited to a certain age group. People of any age can engage in hatha yoga, get in shape, and develop a healthier mental well-being.

Children can learn self-discipline and enhance their physical and mental health at an early age. It has also been indicated that hatha yoga is good for improving memory and concentration and performing the different asanas can provide these perks. Meanwhile, teenagers can improve their flexibility and will make them more resistant to vices and other negative influences that could harm both mind and body (e.g. drugs, drinking). As for older people, the gentleness of hatha yoga compared to other types of yoga will allow mobility and can cure problems regarding poor blood circulation and arthritis. The bottom line is: everyone can enjoy the benefits of mastering hatha yoga as it relieves us many of the issues we suffer through in this modern age.

Since hatha yoga enables relaxation, people also do it before they sleep so as to achieve a peaceful and stable sleep. It aids better working of the mind through meditation. Through deep breathing, it also enhances the body's vitality by the increase of oxygen supply.

There is also lesser risk of injury and muscle strain with hatha yoga even though at times, it can be quite demanding. Unlike traditional forms of exercise such as running on a treadmill, hiking, jogging, and weight training, hatha yoga gives emphasis on the quality of movement instead of quantity. The physical effort required may not be as active and challenging but it can still strengthen your body since poses need to be held for long periods of time.

Hatha yoga doesn't also need a lot of equipment. You don't need to buy a brand-new treadmill or mountain bike to stay in shape. You just have to procure yourself a yoga mat and you are set to go.

Chapter 3   Stretching the Rules Is Not Allowed

Just like any other endeavor, hatha yoga has rules that you have to remember. Observance of these steps that you must accomplish would go a long way to mastering hatha yoga.

Practice with an empty stomach.

It is recommended to refrain from eating two to three hours before a hatha yoga session. The asanas would demand physical contortions of your body as you turn from side to side, twist, and bend forward and backward, among others. Discomfort might be felt during the process if you have not digested your last meal full. However, if you are a person with a fast metabolism, you might end up getting hungry during the session and feel weak because of the lack of food. In this case, you can try to partake in some light back about thirty minutes or an hour before the session.

Listen to Music.

It is advised to listen to soothing music while you are doing your yoga practice. Music would facilitate calming of your mind. Depending on your music choice, an ambience of peace would be achieved. Notice that in meditation sessions or in yoga classes, some of the music that instructors play involves the sounds of nature.

Avoid speaking in the midst of asanas.

Doing asanas is a form of meditation. It is the alternative to sitting still. Unnecessary thoughts are not allowed to enter your mind while you are executing your postures. Talking in the middle of your poses would disrupt your rhythm and would pave the way for distracting ideas to come into your mind. Especially when you are with other people, talking will lead to losing of focus and concentration.

Don't use the restroom during practices.

One must refrain from going to the restroom during your hatha yoga session. The toxins and the water in the body must be worked out in the form of sweat. Furthermore, doing this would interrupt your momentum and rhythm.

Prepare your yoga program beforehand.

Take note that you should not start a yoga session without knowing what asanas you will have to do. Prepare your sequence of asanas and familiarize yourself with the ideal form of each asana. You will not achieve the aims of hatha yoga if you have to stop every after asana in order to look for and decide on the next pose that you must execute. Create your sequence of poses before the practice. Take into consideration the limits of your body and devise a program incorporating the asanas that you will be able to perform during the allotted time that you have given yourself for yoga practice.

Memorize the sequence and arrangement of asanas so you won't have to look into your notes trying to figure out what comes next.

Chapter 4   To-Do List Before Bending

Youjust can't jump straight into hatha yoga without sufficient preparation and equipping yourself with the right materials. Remember that any activity will fail without one planning and getting ready for it first.

What to eat

As I have mentioned, it is not recommended to eat anything before a yoga session. However, during the time when you do eat, there are certain things that you have to bear in mind.

Hatha yoga is basically about strengthening your mind and body. But it will only go a long way into achieving its goal if you do not also exercise other health-beneficial behaviors. For one, you must take note of your diet and the food and beverages that you partake in. Eating processed food, junk food, and other types of food that do not hold nutritional value will cancel out the benefits that hatha yoga can provide. Fresh vegetables and fruits must always be on the menu as they provide the necessary vitamins and minerals needed by the body. Avoid food with excessive fats, proteins, and calories as they are truly detrimental.

Taking in drugs and alcohol goes against the principles of yoga.

What to wear

Do not wear restricting clothes. Tight jeans and shirts would hinder your movements and would not allow you to execute the ideal forms of the asanas. Wear what you are comfortable with. Most people don on yoga pants and loose shirts for maximization of movements. If you can afford not to, do not wear your spectacles during your session. Not only are they in danger of getting damaged while you twist and turn, it would also prove to be distracting if you have to think if they'll fall off of your head while you are doing a certain pose.

What to bring

Whether it is at home or at another avenue, it is best to prepare your own yoga mat that you can lay down on the floor to protect your body from whatever objects are in the floor surface. There are yoga mats that you can buy from the stores available for your perusal.

What to expect

In starting your hatha yoga session, you can expect a slow-paced practice that puts emphasis on the execution of poses and breathing. Expect that at the end of your first session, you might experience soreness in some of your body parts. This is a given since your muscles have just been introduced to a physical activity without prior experience.

Where to practice

Hatha yoga doesn't require any kind of special material or equipment. All you need to do is find a place with a flat surface. You can choose your bedroom or living room or even an empty lounge at your workplace if it's allowed. You can start then by placing your yoga mat on the floor.

Chapter 5   Pose to Turn to a Human Pretzel

There is no proper and fixed sequence of asanas that you must follow. In every yoga class, instructors teach different combinations and sequence of postures. You can actually tailor fit your yoga programs to your abilities and to what you think your body's limits are. Change your program and arrange poses whenever you feel like you are ready to do something harder. As each person is different physically, mentally, and emotionally, do not feel caged by the yoga programs recommended or designed by other people as they may well not be suited for you after all. Create your program with the utmost consideration in order to avoid injury. Don't just throw in recklessly headstands in your program as you may end up breaking your neck. If you feel like you have become more flexible, you can include poses that demands some stretching and headstands later on.

Hatha yoga definitely has an extensive number of postures that you can add in your customized yoga session. As a beginner, you can try to hold these poses for 30 seconds and you may lengthen this time as you practice more.

Moreover, in doing poses from whatever type of yoga, you must remember that you should breathe properly. The usual rule is to inhale when you are stretching your body and exhale when you are contracting your body. Do not be intensely conscious of your breathing. Try to breathe normally and never hold it. You can also try that while exhalation; you say the word *om*.

Mountain Pose

This pose can be used in the beginning or ending of a sequence and can also be utilized as a transition. It is also one of the easiest poses that a beginner can add to his daily program.

Begin by standing on both feet. You have the liberty to either keep your feet together or putting some distance between your feet. Then, extend each of your arms along the sides of your body and tilt your head up slightly.

Butterfly Pose

The butterfly pose starts with sitting down on the floor. Then, carefully bend your knees and situate your feet together in a way that the soles of your right and left foot are touching. Next, pull your heels in or grab your ankles toward your pelvis and press your knees down to the mat. Relax your shoulders and remember to sit up straight. Try to hold the butterfly pose for 30 seconds.

Hero Pose

Begin with sitting on the floor (kneeling style). Your knees must be touching but your feet should be spread a foot apart from each other, enough that your buttocks can rest between them. Your toes should be pointed towards the rear and pressed flat to the yoga mat. Then, stretch your arms upward towards the ceiling and spread your knees as far apart as possible. Next, bend your torso forward so that your chest and abdomen is between your thighs.

Stretch your arms downward towards the floor in front of you and then stretch your head back in order for your chin to rub the floor. Hold on with this pose for 30 seconds.

Knee Head Pose

Sit down on the mat and stretched your legs out in front of you. Then, bend your left knee with your knee caps facing the rear. Keep your right leg straightened out and press the underside of your right knee to the floor. Next, bend your torso forward as far as you can and keep the center of your torso in line with your right leg. Afterwards, stretch out your arms in front of you and extend it as far as you can.

Try to hold this pose for 30 seconds.

Forward Bend

This asana is for stretching and warming up your calves and hips. As the name suggest, forward bends starts with you bending forward at your waist. Let your head, arms, and hand hang heavy in front of you. You can add more tension to the body by holding the backs of your legs with your hands. You can also press your chest as close to your knees as you possibly can.

Plank pose requires exertion of your calves, biceps, triceps, and abdominals most particularly. What you need to do first is lie face down on the mat. Then, lift your body up using your hands and toes to balance yourself. Always remember to keep your body in a straight line. After you do that, tighten your abdominal muscles. At first, you may experience extreme shaking and fatigue in your biceps and triceps that would lead you to lose your balance. But don't you worry about that as it is perfectly normal for a beginner. You need to understand that as you spend more sessions doing this pose, you will notice that you can plan far longer than before.

Downward Dog Pose

This pose, along with the upward dog, is one of the most famous and frequently done asana no matter what type of yoga you are into. Start with planking your body and face down on the mat. Place your palms on the side as if you are doing push-ups. Put one foot of distance between your right and left foot. Inhale then exhale and straighten your arms. Lift your buttocks upwards towards the ceiling and make sure that both your hands and feet are parallel to each other.

Move your chest close towards your knees so that the top of your head will be near the floor. Make sure that your head doesn't really lie on the floor. You can either keep your back straight or you can bend it from the base of your spine to make it look concave.

Try to hold this pose for 1 minute. Your gaze must be concentrated beyond your feet.

From the downward facing dog pose, you can then proceed to the next posture, which is the upward facing dog. Be sure you are ready for this.

Upward Dog Pose

With the upward dog pose, your body will resemble the opposite of downward dog pose. In this pose, begin by lying flat on your stomach with your feet distanced by one foot or so. Place your palms at each side of your body and your toes should be pointed straight towards the rear.

During an exhalation, raise your torso upward by pulling your arms forward and straightening it. Keep your legs flat on the mat and locked at the knees. Then, proceed to bending from your lower back region and raise your upper torso and shoulders upwards towards the ceiling.

As far as you can, stretch your head back.

Tree Pose

Stand with your feet slightly apart. Then, lift your right leg and bend it at the knee. Point your right foot towards your left thigh. Rest your right foot either above or below the knee. Do not place your right foot exactly on your knee as it would not provide any kind of physical challenge. Balance yourself on your current position and extend your arms above your head.

Warrior Two

There are three types of warrior poses but hatha yoga, more often than not, incorporates warrior two since it is a good transitional pose between asanas. This pose would require effort on the part of your arms, legs, and thighs. What you need to do first is to stand with your feet firmly placed together. Bend your right leg until it will form a ninety degree angle to the ground. Then, with your left leg this time, slide it back until it sticks or angles out straight behind you. Afterwards, turn your torso slightly to the left while extending your arms on each side of your body. The direction of your head should be towards the front of the room.

Extended Three Angle Pose

This asana requires effort of your leg muscles, resulting to being toned and strengthened. As it requires you to twist your body, it would relieve backaches. Start with standing with your feet together, toes and ankles touching. Inhale and during exhalation, you must spread your feet part up to a distance of three feet. They should be parallel to each other. Then, extend your arms to the side with your palms facing downward. Your head should be facing front.

Then, turn your right foot ninety degrees to the right while turning your left foot just slightly to the right as well. Next, bend your trunk or torso horizontally to the right and place your right hand on your right ankle. If you can, you can also try to place your right hand on the floor next to your right foot.

Meanwhile, extend your left hand upward towards the ceiling with your left arm straight. Extend or stretch the back of your neck and then turn your head as far to the left as possible and stare up past your outstretched left hand. Hold this position.

Half ship pose

This specific pose will target your abdominal muscles and your back. Start by sitting on the floor. Then, place your hands behind your head and interlock your fingers. Place your legs together with your kneecaps and ankles touching. Then, recline your torso backwards to an angle of about forty-five degrees until both your feet starts to rise off of the floor. Raise your legs until your feet are in the same height or level with your head. You must make sure that the weight of your body is resting on your buttocks and not on the lower part of your spine as it would be harmful if you do the latter. Try to hold this position for 30 seconds to 1 minute.

Entire boat posture

Like the half ship pose, the entire boat pose will help you strengthen your abdominal and back muscles. It will also help in the reduction of fat around your waist. The very first thing you need to do is to sit on the floor. Keep your palms by your side and with your legs straightened out. Then, recline your torso backwards and raise your legs until both your feet are a foot higher compared to your head. The ankles of your feet should be touching each other. The challenge now lies on balancing your weight on your buttocks so that no part of your lower spine is touching the mat.

As with your arms, extend them straight past your knees. They should be parallel to the floor with the palms faced towards each other. Hold this pose for 30 seconds if you can.

Locust Pose

The locust pose relies heavily on the movement of the abdominal and leg muscles as well as some parts of your back area. Begin this pose by lying face down on your mat with your ankles touching each other and your hands by your side. Then, raise your head, chest, and legs all at the same time as high as you possibly can off the floor. Meanwhile, your arms should be extended straight towards the rear.

Hold this position for a minute and afterwards, lower your head, chest, and feet to the floor slowly.

Intense Stretch Pose

Begin by standing straight. Lift your arms over your head and stretch them towards the ceiling. Next, swing your arms and torso downward so you can place your palms down on the mat. Put your palms on the mat behind you as far as you can so that your chest is pressed closely against your thighs. Then, place your head on your shins.

Hold this pose for upto 5 minutes while breathing fully.

Camel posture

This pose requires the backward stretching of your spine. It demands a kind of flexibility in order to maneuver this move. First, you have to kneel on the mat with your thighs and feet touching each other. Proceed to placing your palms on your hips. The thumbs of your hands must be touching your lower spine. Next, curve your torso backwards and then place your palms on your feet. Make sure that your palms on your soles. At the same time, stretch your chest forward.

With your palms on your feet, stretch your head back as far as you possibly can. Hold this pose for 30 seconds.

Corpse Pose

The corpse pose may be one of the favorite poses of yoga enthusiasts. Most sessions end with a corpse pose since it provides you a chance to rest. The degree of immobility will relax your mind and body. All you need to do is lie on your back on a firm surface. Keep your body in a straight line and spread your arms at an angle of forty-five degrees with your palms turned upward.

Relax your jaw enough that your upper and lower teeth are touching each other just slightly. Additionally, don't tense up your tongue.

Extend your legs, as well. Try to relax and focus your mind into your breathing and the beating of your heart. Don't think about anything else. Engage in heavy breathing for one minute and then slow down the rate of your breathing until no air is felt moving through your nostrils.

Let your breathing take the wayward thoughts out of your mind.

Chapter 6   Memos for a Yogi

What you need to realize right from the start is that you cannot expect your body to respond to the demands of hatha yoga immediately. And always bear that in mind. It needs time to cope with the new experience that you are introducing to it. Do not be discouraged if you can't instantly perform the sequence of asanas provided. Hatha yoga takes some deal of time and effort on your part.

As for the best time to practice the asanas, itis recommended to do it during the early morning when both your body and mind have rested and are free from fatigue. The conditions in the morning will boost your determination to perform the asanas and it will also give you the necessary strength. Daily practice is ideal for one to reap the benefits from hatha yoga. Especially when you are just beginning, you must allot some time every day to doing yoga in your home. As for the postures that you must execute, newbies should start first with the basics so as to not surprise your body. And that is a must. As you advance, you may work on more complicated and demanding postures. You can also opt to lengthen the time you spend for practice from just 20 minutes per day to even an hour in order to maximize the potential hatha yoga can give.

It is also recommended that you empty your bowels and bladder before you start your session as their state may affect your concentration during the session.

There are also precautions that you must take. You should take a leave from doing yoga when you are suffering through painful health complications. People with fever, migraine, menstrual cramps, etc. should refrain from engaging in the physical activities demanded by hatha yoga as they may worsen one's condition.

As what was mentioned before, you will definitely have some problems and difficulty when it comes to holding your postures for the ideal length of time. You may find yourself even incapable of remaining upright and balanced in some of the poses. But with more practice, you will surely achieve and accomplish those poses. Hard work is needed in hatha yoga. You can't expect results when you don't try in the first place. Don't ever over-exert yourself. Remember that damaging your body will never be one of the purposes of hatha yoga.

In order to avoid injury, take note of your body. Be wary of any pain that you may feel. Back off and stop your postures whenever you feel an unbearable, acute pain.

And most importantly, include hatha yoga in your lifestyle because you want it there. Don't do it just because you're pressured by what other people are saying or just for the fun of it. Hatha yoga needs serious dedication and commitment for without them, you would probably stop after only just a session. Bear in mind the benefits it can give you and enjoy the whole process. You have all the chance to find comfort and joy in doing hatha yoga as you are not competing with other people. You are only competing with yourself; you're testing your limits and breaking through the boundaries of your mind and body. Remember that you are doing hatha yoga in order to achieve a better you and treat this as a strong motivation to continue no matter what happens.

Conclusion

Thank you again for downloading this book!

I hope this book was able to help you to understand what hatha yoga truly is and realize that it is a very good stepping stone towards the practice of yoga, take note of the mental and physical benefits that it can provide you, remember the rules that you must abide by, and bear in mind the step-by-step guide provided with regards to the different asanas of hatha yoga.

Once you've completed this book in full, the next step is to prepare yourself to officially start becoming a yogi. Acquire the necessary materials that you need and ready your mind and body. Remember the things that you must do while you are executing the asanas and take into consideration the precautions that you must heed. Most especially, take this new journey towards a healthier lifestyle with determination and dedication.

Finally, if you enjoyed this book, please take the time to share your thoughts and post a review on Amazon. It'd be greatly appreciated!

In addition please be sure to take a look on the next page as I have provided you with more high quality books I've published which I'm certain can help you out a ton!

Thank you and good luck on your journey!

Bonus Chapter: Morning Yoga Poses

As discussed, some poses are designed to bring energy flow and help you start your day. These poses should be done in the morning. If you can, do them as soon as you rise. Some people need time to hit the snooze, get a cup of coffee and feel human before doing anything. That's fine too, but remember that these poses can actually help you wake up and start your day.

Back Bends

Back bends should only be done in the morning. They are very invigorating and will give you a lot of energy. These backbend poses are actually very easy to do, even for the beginner yogi.

1. Bow Pose (Dhanurasana)

Start by laying on your stomach with your arms at your sides, palms up. Breathe deeply, in and out. As you breathe out, bend your knees up until your heels are as close to your buttocks as possible. Breathe in. Breathe out, brining your hands up to grasp your ankles. Breathe in. Breathe out and lift your heels away from your buttocks, while also lifting your thighs off of the floor. This will naturally bring your torso up from the floor without straining the back.

You are now in the bow pose. This pose can make it difficult to breathe because your stomach is pressed against the floor. Make sure you continue to take measured breaths, in and out, and only hold the pose for about 30 seconds.

2. Bridge Pose (Setubandha)

Begin by lying on the floor on your back, legs straight and arms to your sides, palms down. Breathe in and out in measured breaths. Breathe out and bend your knees, placing your feet on the floor as close to your buttocks as possible. Breathe in. Breathing out, press your feet and arms into the floor, lifting your buttocks off of the floor. Continue your deep breathing. Bring your arms underneath you and clasp your hands, still pressing them into the floor. This provides additional support for your shoulders to lift from the floor.

Continue raising your buttocks until your thighs are about parallel to the floor. Raise your pubis toward the navel, lengthening the tailbone and pushing your knees away from your hips. Exhale as you lift your chin and bring it away from the chest, broaden your shoulder blades, and lift them until your chin meets the torso. You should do this in one fluid movement if possible.

You are now in the bridge pose. You can hold this pose up to one minute. Remember to continue deep breathing while in the pose. When complete, exhale while rolling the spine slowly to the floor.

3. Cobra Pose (Bhujanga)

Start by lying on the floor on your stomach. The tops of your feet, your legs and thighs and your pelvis should be firmly pressed against the floor. Place your hands on the floor in line with your shoulders, elbows pressed in toward your body. Breathe in and straighten your arms slowly to raise your chest off of the floor. Make sure you keep your feet, legs and pelvis firmly pressed to the floor. Breathe deeply while you firm your shoulder blades toward your back and push your side ribs forward. Do not push the front ribs forward because this will strain your back. Continue breathing easily while you hold the pose for about 30 seconds.

4. Cow Pose (Bitilasana)

Begin by getting on your hands on knees, knees placed even with the hips, arms even with the shoulders, hands pressed to the floor, and the tops of the feet pressed to the floor. This is called the "table top" position. Breathe in while lifting both your buttocks and tailbone and your chest upward. Your belly will naturally drop toward the floor. Hold this position for about 30 seconds. You can release and repeat up to 20 times. Each time you bend you should inhale, and each time you release you should exhale.

5. Fish Pose (Matsyasana)

Start by laying on your back with legs stretched out, arms at your sides with palms pressing the floor. Draw your knees up so that your feet are firmly on the floor. Begin your deep breathing. Breathing in, lift your pelvis off of the floor and place your hands beneath your buttocks and tuck in your elbows. On another breath in, press your forearms and elbows against the floor. Again on an inhale, raise your torso and head up. Release your neck and allow your head to come back down to the floor slowly. Depending on the arch of your back your head may rest on the floor on the back or the crown. Do not place weight on your head so that your neck does not get crunched by pressure. On an exhale lower your legs flat against the floor, toes pointing up. Stay in this position for up to 30 seconds, then release and lower your torso back to the floor while breathing out.

6. Locust Pose (Salabhasana)

Lie on your stomach, forehead touching the floor, arms at your sides, palms up. Rotate your thighs inward by turning your big toes toward each other. While breathing out lift your upper body and legs off of the floor so that you are resting on your lower ribs and pelvis. Raise your arms until they are parallel to the floor and reach back. Firm the buttocks and legs and reach back toward your feet. Raise your head to look forward or slightly upward, but don't crunch the back of your neck. Hold this position for up to one minute, then slowly release on an exhale.

7. Sphinx Pose

Lay down on your stomach with your legs next to each other, the tops of your feet resting on the floor, and your arms out in front of you. Turn your toes toward each other and roll your thighs inward so that you are lengthening your spine. Pull your arms up lifting yourself off of the floor, your hands pressed to the floor and your arms parallel to each other and elbows bent. Slowly raise yourself up, stretching your legs back as if you are going to press the wall with your feet to further lengthen the spine. Once in the mild back bend your arms should be at a 90 degree angle, and you should be facing forward. Breathe deeply for about 10 breaths, then slowly ease your upper body back to the floor on an exhale.

8. Upward Facing Dog Pose (Urdhva Mukha Svanasana)

Lay down on the floor on your stomach, stretch out your legs and place the tops of your feet on the floor. Your elbows should be slightly bent with your hands pressed against the floor to position your forearms parallel with the floor. Turn your thighs inward and firm your buttocks. Push up a bit with your hands as if you are going to scoot yourself forward along the floor. On an inhale straighten your arms and lift up your upper torso and legs slightly simultaneously. Press your tailbone toward the pelvis. Firm your shoulder blades against your back and lift your upper torso further. You should not push the front ribs forward or you could hurt your back, and you should also take care not to crunch your neck as you look forward. Hold this position for up to one minute, and release on an exhale.

Standing Poses

Standing poses build strength and stamina. They are good to do in the morning or in the afternoon, but should not be done at night. These poses also give you a sense of grounding because your feet are planted firmly on the floor. All of these poses will have you starting by standing upright with your feet planted on the floor, arms to your sides and facing forward.

9. Big Toe Pose (Padangusthasana)

This pose is about lengthening and strengthening your body. Start by tightening your thighs, which will lift your kneecaps. Keep your legs completely straight as you bend at the hip to touch your toes. Grasp your big toes with your first finger and thumb wrapped around. If you cannot touch your toes, place a strap beneath and in the center of your feet before you begin and grab these straps when you bend down. Press your toes down. Straighten your elbows as if you are going to stand back up, which will lengthen your torso. Lift your buttocks slowly as you take pressure off of your legs and loosen the hamstrings. Bend your elbows out to your sides and pull up on your toes (or the strap). This will allow you to stretch safely into a deep forward bend. Hold this pose for about one minute, then release your toes or strap and slowly swing your head and torso upright while taking a deep breath.

10. Chair Pose (Utkatasana)

Taking a deep breath in, raise your arms parallel to the floor. Keep them parallel to each other with palms facing inward. As you breathe out, bend your knees until your thighs are as close to parallel to the floor as possible. Your buttocks will point out, your knees will be over the feet (but don't bring your knees past your toes to avoid knee injury or strain), and your upper body will be slightly bent forward to create a 90 degree angle with your thighs. Press your thighs toward your heels, lengthen your back, and bring your arms up, hands pointing straight above you. Hold this pose for up to one minute. Inhale while straightening your knees and coming out of the position, reaching up through your arms to bring yourself back to a standing position.

11. Extended Side Angle Pose (Utthita Parsvakonasana)

Step (or jump) your feet until they are about four feet apart. Raise your arms, palms down, until they are parallel to the floor. Turn your feet, your left foot slightly to the right and your right foot to the right in a 90 degree angle. Your heels should be evenly aligned. Next, turn your right thigh to the outside, putting your knee in line with your ankle. In one fluid motion rotate your left hip to the right and forward and your upper torso to the left and back. Ground your left heel to the floor for balance. Carefully bend your right knee over your right ankle until your shin is perpendicular to the floor and bring the thigh as close to parallel with the floor as possible. Turn the palm of your left hand toward your body and lift your arm up toward the ceiling. Extend your left arm over your ear while bending to touch your right ankle with your fingertips or palm. You can hold this pose for up to one minute. To come out of the pose press down on your heels to ground and slowly come out of the pose, lengthening your arm toward the ceiling and back down to assist your body in coming out of the bend. Repeat this pose with the other side.

12. Extended Triangle Pose (Utthita Trikonasana)

Place your feet about four feet apart. Lift your arms, palms down, until your arms are at your sides parallel to the floor. Turn your left foot inward to the right and your right foot to the right in a 90 degree angle. Your heels should be evenly aligned. Turn your right thigh to the outside, putting your knee in line with your ankle. Breathing out, bend at the hip to extend your upper body down and to the right over the plane of the right leg, then rotate your upper body to the left. Finally, rest your right hand on your right shin or ankle and bring your left arm up until your hand points to the ceiling. Remain in this pose for up to one minute, then breathe in planting your heels firmly on the floor and stretching your arm toward the ceiling to slowly come out of the bend and come upright.

13. High Lunge

Stand and bend forward at the hips. Breathing in take your left foot back with the ball of your foot on the floor for balance. Your right knee should be at a 90 degree angle. Bending forward, lay your torso on your right thigh while firming your left thigh and pressing it up toward the ceiling. Bring your arms down and press your fingertips to the floor for balance. Keep your left leg straight and stretch your heel toward the floor. To come out of the lunge Breathe out and move your right foot back to beside your left and slowly come out of the forward bend.

Printed in Great Britain
by Amazon.co.uk, Ltd.,
Marston Gate.